The Best Hair Care Remedies to Embrace

A Comprehensive Recipe Book on Improving and Having Healthy Hair

By

Angel Burns

License Notices

This book or parts thereof might not be reproduced in any format for personal or commercial use without the written permission of the author. Possession and distribution of this book by any means without said permission is prohibited by law.

All content is for entertainment purposes and the author accepts no responsibility for any damages, commercially or personally, caused by following the content.

Table of Contents

Chapter 1: Introduction

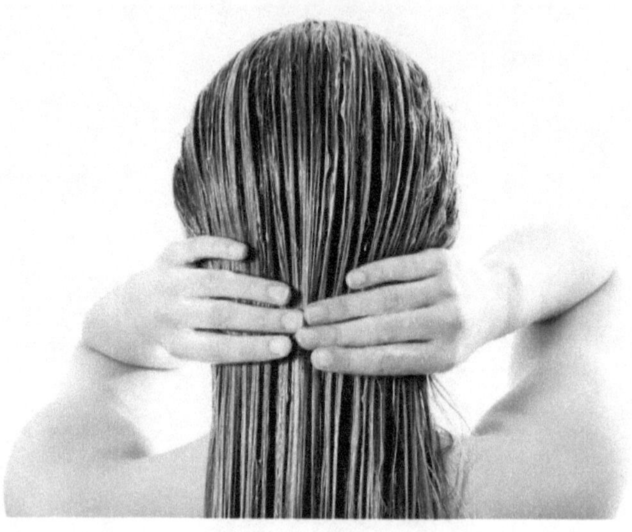

Hair grows from follicles all over the scalp. Hair cells are some of the fastest-growing cells in the body. Each person is born with all the hair follicles they will ever have, about five million of them. The follicle grows from beneath the skin of the scalp and is sometimes referred to as a bulb, because that is what it looks like. Look at a tulip bulb. It is a rounded teardrop shape and usually has several sheaths coming from the small top. That is exactly what a hair follicle looks like.

The shape of the hair follicle determines what kind of hair a person has. Round follicles produce straight hair while oval ones send forth curly hair. If you have round follicles today, it doesn't necessarily mean you will have them for life. They can change shape throughout your life.

Each person normally has about 100,000 hair strands on his head. The hair shaft is made up of three layers. The hair cuticle is the outside layer that protects two other inner layers.

The hair cuticles are flat and they reflect light. So, if you have shiny hair, it is an indication that each strand is healthy. When hair cuticles are flat, they overlap and protect the inner layers from different elements such as heat from the sun, dust, chlorine and other chemicals.

When the hair cuticles are not healthy or are damaged, they do not overlap tightly. They separate causing the hair to become dry. This dryness can also cause the inner layers to become dry. This further causes the hair to look dull and break easily.

Hair has natural oil, called sebum, which protects it and makes it shiny. Protecting your hair by caring for it will play a major role in its health and appearance.

There are different hair types. Some people have curly hair, others have straight hair. Some hairs are naturally dry while some are very fine. Regardless of the type of hair you have, you have to care for it gently. Hair care should depend on the type of hair that you have, your lifestyle and your style preferences.

People who have dry or curly hair will need more care in comparison to people with straight or fine hair. Some people's hairs are oilier than others, especially when they are teenagers. The sebaceous glands are known to be overactive and result in production of more sebum on the skin, scalp and hair. Oil can clog pores and follicles.

Hair care is also dependent on a person's interests and levels of activity. For people who are always at the beach, the hair is exposed to too much sun's heat and other harmful particles. You may not have to wash your hair too often. For active people or those engaged in a lot of sports, hair may easily get dry or oily. It is better to wash it frequently.

Hair styling can also be a determining factor for hair care. The use of curling irons, straightening irons, and other chemical cosmetic products may either be useful or harmful, which makes it necessary to provide your strands with proper care.

Not all hairstyling chemicals will work for all types of hair. Here are some important tips regarding chemical treatments.

Straighteners or relaxers are used to break bonds in chemical bonds when a person has curly hair. It normally contains lye, which may cause irritation in the skin as well as hair breakage. Be sure to use relaxers the right way. Mix them in appropriate amounts and leave them on your hair at the proper time periods. Before you get a relaxing treatment, make sure that you do not brush, comb or scratch your hair or you may increase the risk of breakage and irritation.

If you want to get another relaxing or straightening treatment, you should only do so after at least 6 to 8 weeks. You do not want chemical build-up on your hair follicles and you only need to treat the new growths.

Perming treatments. This is the opposite of straighteners. Perms result into curly hair. Both chemicals pose the same risks of irritation and breakage.

Hair color or dye. There are two kinds of dyes: permanent and semi-permanent. Permanent hair colors stay with your strands until they grow. Semi-permanent colors will fade away after some washings. Henna is a kind of semi-permanent hair dye. Be sure to check your skin for irritation before having dyes applied. Always go for a patch test.

Some dangers posed by hair dyes are the following: burning, irritation, redness, hair loss and allergic reactions. Hair dyes should not be used on eyebrows or eyelashes.

Problems related to the Hair

Whatever style of hair you may have, you cannot escape having a bad hair day at one point in your life.

Below, we focus on a number of known hair problems that men and women alike suffer from every day if not at one point in their life.

- Dry, brittle hair is due to the lack of moisture in your hair can lead to other hair problems like split ends, falling hair or frizzy hair. This is normally caused by prolonged exposure to heat like the sun or electric styling tools.

- Limp hair, other than medical related reason is also caused by hair care products build up. If you are using shampoo or conditioner that is heavy on the hair, this will build up over time making your hair lifeless and without volume.

- Split ends are the most common hair problem. When your hair becomes dry and brittle, the hair cuticle is damaged, causing the ends to split. Excessive hair styling, blow drying, hair coloring and straightening are some of the major causes of split ends

- Dandruff and flaky scalp cause itchiness. Your scalp is where your hair is rooted. It is the bed of your hair and it needs proper washing and care just as much as your hair. The overuse of hair care products with lots of chemicals can cause the skin on your scalp to dry leaving flakes to form. Lack of nutrients can also cause your scalp to get dry.

- Dull hair is due to lack of moisture in your hair. Lack of protein, vitamins, and minerals from eating the right food can cause to the lack of natural moisture and shine of your hair. Chemical build-up from hair care products can also cause your hair to become dull and limp.

- Heat damaged hair is caused by prolonged exposure to the sun and the excessive use of blow dryer. No matter how healthy your hair is, excessive exposure to heat can cause your hair to become dry and brittle. Eventually, this could lead to other hair problems.

- Gray hair appears as part of the signs of aging. But, younger folks may exhibit gray hair, too. Exposure to heat, smoke, dirt, and chemicals can cause your hair to get damaged and become gray. Inadequate essential minerals and vitamins can result into gray hair. Medical conditions that require radiation treatment is also known to cause gray hair.

Falling Hair or Hair Loss is another common problem. Falling hair is caused by using the wrong hair care product and unhealthy scalp. If you are under chemotherapy treatment, hair loss occurs due to the exposure to radiation. Other health conditions that can cause hair loss includes alopecia, severe infections, surgery and, using of antidepressants.

Chapter 2: Why use DIY Solutions

I know you may feel like making your own hair products can be time-consuming. We love convenience. The convenience of just going to the store. But your tresses need tender loving care, one that many store-bought hair care products simply cannot give. If you love your hair and want to give it the care it deserves, then spare some time for making your own homemade hair care treatments.

Making your own natural hair products may seem like a lot of work. But you will like the results. With this said, below is a list of the topnotch benefits of making your own natural hair care concoctions.

1. You get to find the right mix to target specific hair issues

Do you think conventional hair products have the right ingredients to properly nourish your natural hair? Do you think they are your best options? If you have been using certain products for a while and you are still suffering from hair dryness then you are probably mistaken. The truth is these store-bought hair products are commonly loaded with hair drying chemicals. Many promise you the world when it comes to caring for your tresses, but they may actually do more damage than you can imagine.

On the other hand, making your own mix of hair care products gives you an upper hand. You can handpick the ingredients to make sure they are all natural. Natural ingredients won't cause damage to your hair as long as you use them wisely. You can target specific hair issues by carefully choosing the best ingredients to reach your goals.

If you want to moisturize your hair for instance, you can go for nourishing ingredients such as Aloe Vera, extra virgin olive oil, honey, egg, coconut milk and oil and a whole lot more. If your natural hair could use some shine, take advantage of the shining properties of avocado oil, castor oil and apple cider vinegar. If you want more defined curls, use flaxseed gel, mango butter, Shea butter and beeswax.

There are thousands of combinations and mixtures you can come up with. The secret is to know what your hair craves and deliver with the best natural ingredients you can get your hands on.

2. Save money saving your hair

Although there are now more organic natural hair products on the market, the problem is they can be expensive.

Save your wallet and save your hair making your own natural mixture. Most of these ingredients are readily available. They may actually sit right in your kitchen.

Making your own natural hair care products does not have to cost you an arm and a leg. It is a matter of making use of what you can easily find. And there are a lot. You just need to discover them. And when you do, make sure to take advantage!

3. It requires little effort

Another great advantage of making your own hair care potions is that they do not require that much effort. Some may need more work. But most of these homemade recipes can be prepared in less than 15 minutes.

You do not even have to be a mix-tress or a genius to make one. You just have to pay attention and keep learning.

The Best Ingredients to Use for Homemade Hair Treatment Solutions

Are you ready to turn things around and make a glorious change in the name of your crowning glory? Read on to find out what natural potions you can create in the comforts of your kitchen!

But heading to the recipes, we'll take a look at some of the best ingredients to use making your own natural hair product.

Avocado

Known as a superfood, avocado is not just good for making guacamole or smoothie, they also offer loads of benefits for your natural hair. For instance, this fruit is rich in vitamins A, B, D and E. These nutrients help prevent the escape of moisture and makes the hair shiny. On top of that, avocado can also strengthen brittle hair so you do not have to worry about split ends. To make shampoo, you can mash avocado or add avocado oil with other fantastic natural ingredients.

Banana

The most common problem with natural hair is manageability. Hair can be very dry. If you have been using conventional shampoo all this time then it should not be any surprise. But banana can fix that.

Added to your shampoo recipe, banana can help protect as well as soften your kinks, coils and curls. It gives your hair the shine it needs and at the same time, strengthen it so breakage and split ends are prevented.

Coconut

Known for its moisturizing properties, coconut milk and coconut oil are also helpful in promoting hair growth. Do you have dandruff? Coconut can fix that too while leaving your hair smelling like tropical breeze.

Olive Oil

Dryness is a common problem with hair. Extra virgin olive oil prevents that from happening. Add extra virgin olive oil to your basic shampoo recipe so you can shine out your strands as well as prevent hair loss.

Almond Oil

This natural ingredient does more than make a homemade shampoo smell great. In fact, it can smoothen out hair cuticles that can help prevent hair shedding. It is just a bonus that it smells sweet and delicious.

There are plenty of excellent natural ingredients you can use to make your own shampoo concoction. Note these superfoods for added benefits.

Chapter 3: Recipes

DIY Organic Honey Shampoo

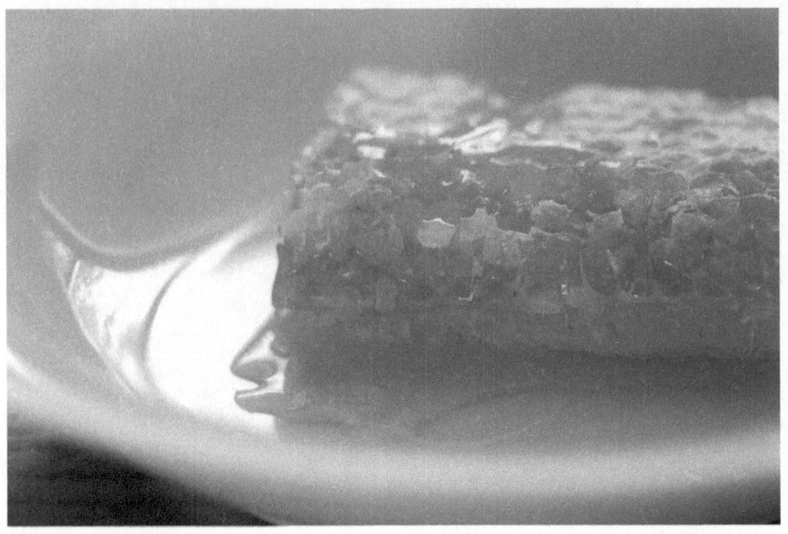

Ingredients:

- Chamomile.
- 6 tbsps. water, warm.
- 2 tbsps. honey, raw.
- Carrot seed oil.

Directions:

1. First, heat your honey and water together on low heat until it is just barely melting.

2. Stir the honey and water to combine them and then remove from stove top.

3. If you wish to preserve more of your honey's natural nutrients, you can heat the water first and then combine it with the honey.

4. Add your favorite organic essential oils and use like regular shampoo.

5. Note that the mixture will be watery – this is how it should be.

6. Pour the shampoo in an unbreakable container and keep near the shower.

7. The proper ratio is 3 tablespoons of water for every 1 tablespoon of organic honey.

Organic Shikakai and Reetha DIY Shampoo

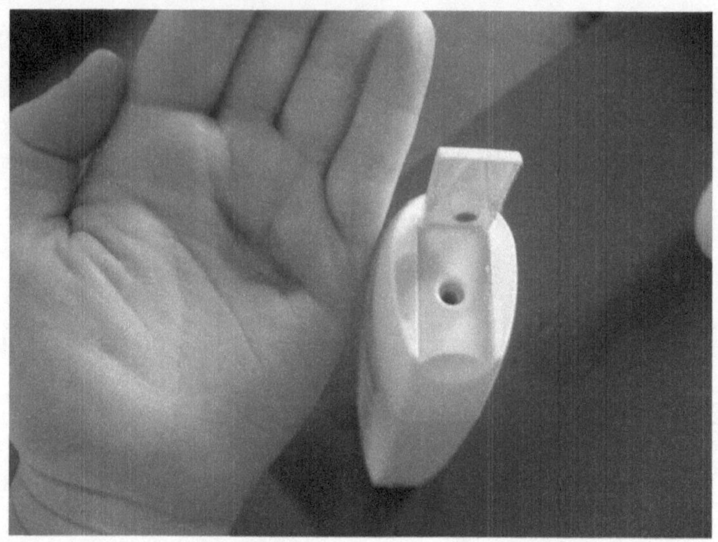

Ingredients:

- 1 c. organic reetha
- 2 tsps. organic Shikakai powder

Directions:

1. Soak the organic reetha in water and leave it overnight. The next morning, pour water and reetha into your blender. Add the organic Shikakai powder and then blend until the mixture is smooth.

2. Use as you would a conventional shampoo. You may leave this organic shampoo in your hair just a bit longer, and then rinse with warm water.

DIY Organic High Protein Egg Shampoo

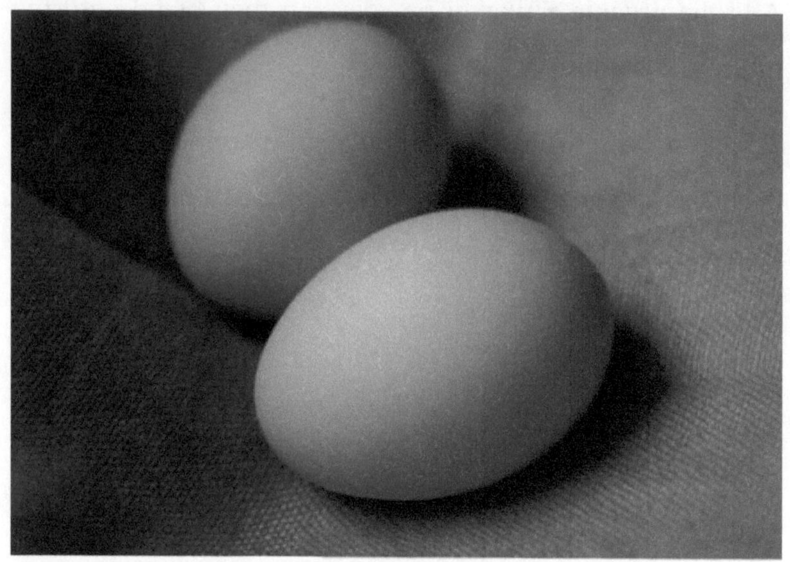

Ingredients:

- 1 tbsp. Shikakai powder, organic
- 2 eggs, free range
- 1 tsp. olive oil, organic
- 1 tsp. Aloe Vera, organic
- 4 drops, organic peppermint
- 1 tbsp. Cassia, organic
- 1 tsp. honey, organic
- 1 tsp. Amla powder, organic

Directions:

1. Crack two eggs in a bowl. Whisk them together thoroughly.

2. Add essential oils if you are using them. Mix well.

3. You may add 2-4 tablespoons of warm water to your mixture. If you have already oiled your hair or your hair is naturally greasy, do not dilute the shampoo.

DIY Organic African Black Soap Shampoo

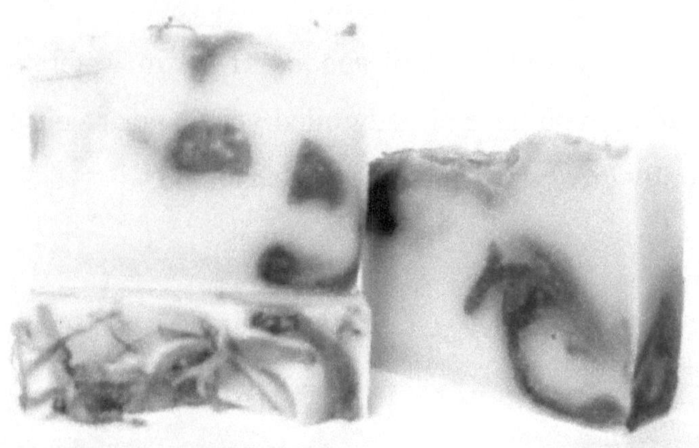

Ingredients:

- 2 tbsps. organic honey, raw.
- 4 tbsps. organic African Black soap, crumbled.
- 1 c. water, hot
- 3 tbsps. organic grapeseed oil

Directions:

1. Mix your ingredients in a lidded jar or plastic bottle.

2. Shake the container well and let it cool for 15-20 minutes before using. When it has cooled somewhat, the consistency will be thicker, and easier to apply to your hair. The hair will also be able to utilize the shampoo better when it is thicker.

3. Use just one-half this mixture for washing your hair. Cover and save the remainder for the next time you wash your hair.

4. It will take time for your hair to become accustomed to the healthy, organic ingredients. Don't expect to see miraculous results after just a few days.

5. If the shampoo doesn't feel as though it is completely rinsed from your hair, rinse your hair with vinegar to clear it out.

DIY Organic Avocado Homemade Shampoo for Treating Oily Hair

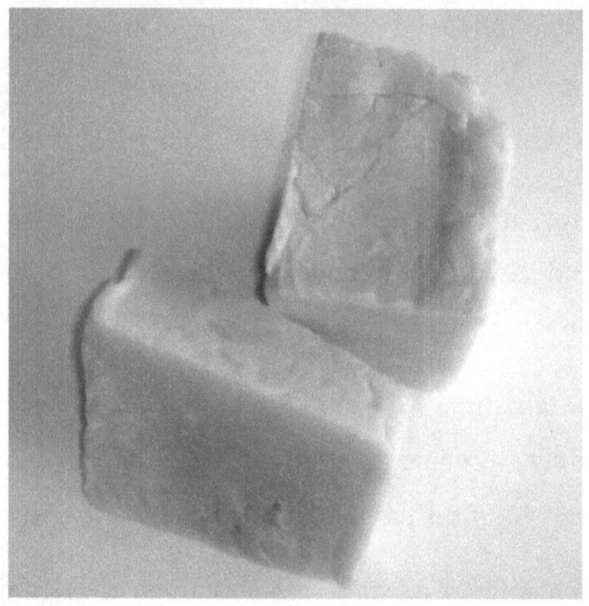

Ingredients:

- 1 organic peeled and pitted avocado, ripe
- 2 tsps. baking soda
- ¼ c. distilled water, warm

Directions:

1. Blend your ingredients until you have a smooth consistency, like paste. Apply as you would your old shampoo and rinse well.

DIY Organic Apple Cider Vinegar Shampoo

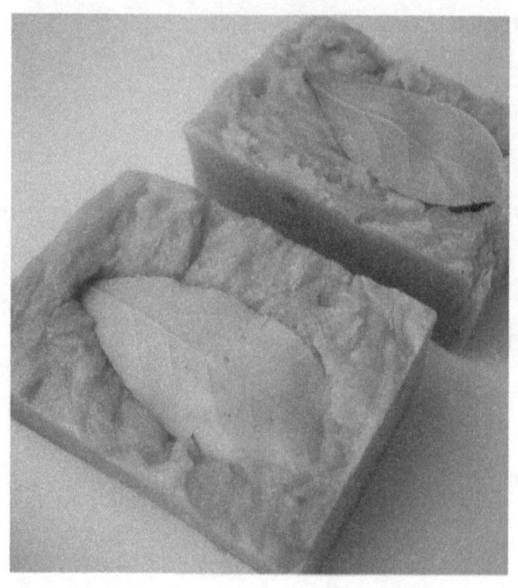

Ingredients:

- 2 tbsps. organic lemon juice, fresh
- 1 tsp. organic apple cider vinegar
- 1 oz. organic olive oil
- 1 egg, free range

Directions:

1. Toss your organic ingredients in a blender. Blend until the mixture is smooth.

2. Apply the mixture like a shampoo and massage for several minutes.

3. Rinse well with warm water.

Organic Lemon & Coconut DIY Shampoo

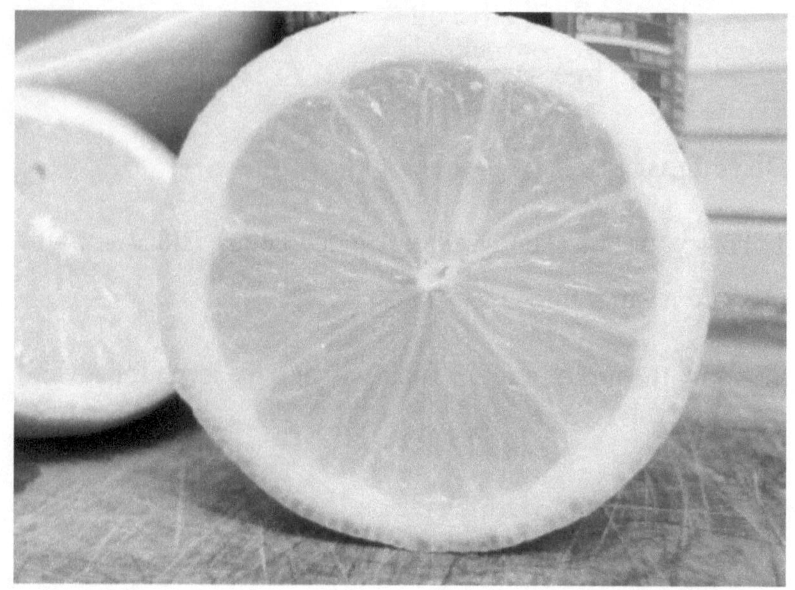

Ingredients:

- 1 c. organic castile soap, liquid
- 1 tbsp. organic coconut oil
- 20 drops organic essential oil, lemongrass

Directions:

1. Pour castile soap in a bowl.

2. Add your organic coconut oil. Stir thoroughly,

3. Add 20 drops of organic lemongrass essential oil,

4. Combine the mixture again.

Homemade Organic Anti-Dandruff Shampoo

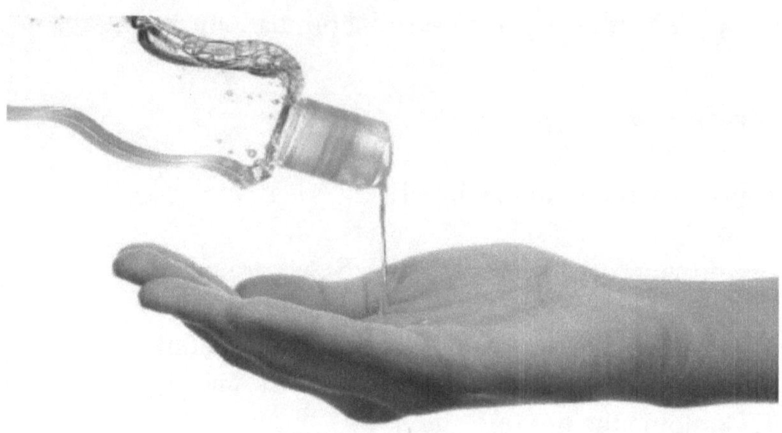

Ingredients:

- ¼ c. organic vegetable glycerin
- 2 tsps. organic coconut oil
- ¼ c. organic coconut milk
- 4 drops organic essential oil, geranium
- ½ c. organic castile soap, liquid

Directions:

1. Combine your ingredients, mixing well and then pouring into the container you'll be using. You can use old shampoo bottles if you like, or empty bottles sold at DIY cosmetic stores.

2. Apply as you would conventional shampoo, and rinse well.

DIY Organic Coconut Dry Hair Shampoo

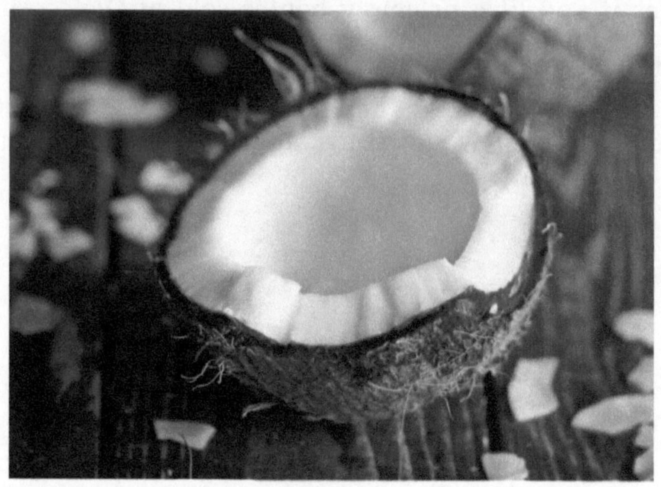

Ingredients:

- ¼ c. coconut milk
- 1 tbsp. organic almond oil
- 10 drops organic essential oil

Directions:

1. Mix all your ingredients and shake the bottle well. If it is too runny, you can add baking soda to thicken it up.

2. Wash as usual and rinse.

Organic Castile Soap DIY Shampoo

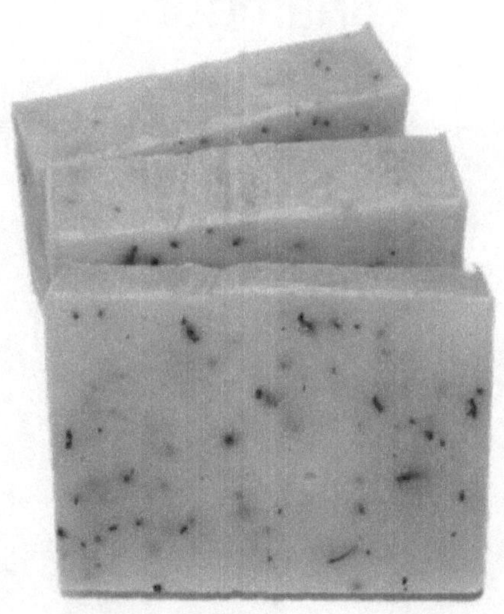

Ingredients:

- 2 tbsps. organic apple cider vinegar
- 1 tbsp. organic tea tree oil
- ¼ c. water, warm
- 1 c. organic castile soap

Directions:

1. Mix ingredients together and then pour the mixture into a bottle.

2. Add several drops of your preferred organic essential oil.

DIY Organic Stinging Nettle Shampoo

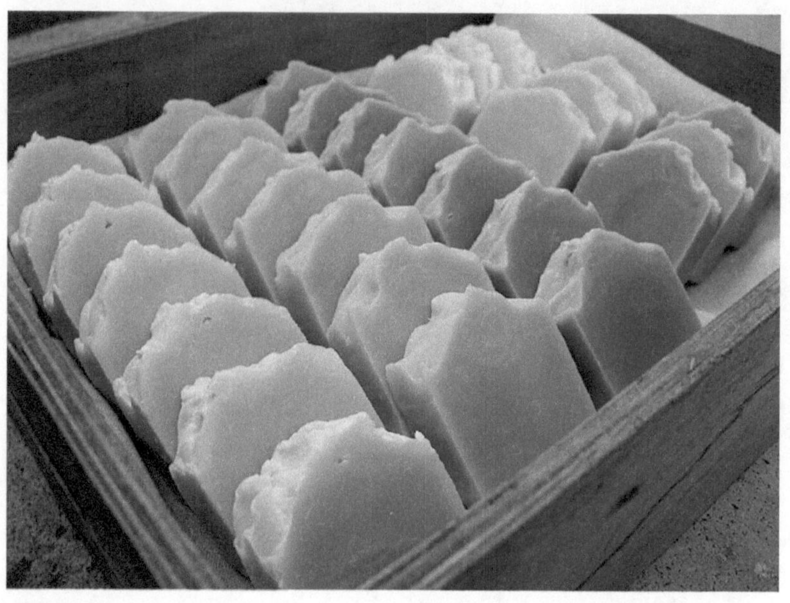

Ingredients:

- 16 oz. organic nettle shampoo
- 3 vials organic vitamin B complex
- ¾ oz. organic stinging nettle extract
- 1 ¾ oz. castor oil

Directions:

1. Combine ingredients together. Use glass containers so that plastic and herbs don't interact.

2. Use to improve the overall condition of your damaged hair and to prevent it from thinning.

3. New hair growth will be visible after about four weeks or so of steady use. Continue using for three to four more months.

Organic Oatmeal DIY Dry Shampoo

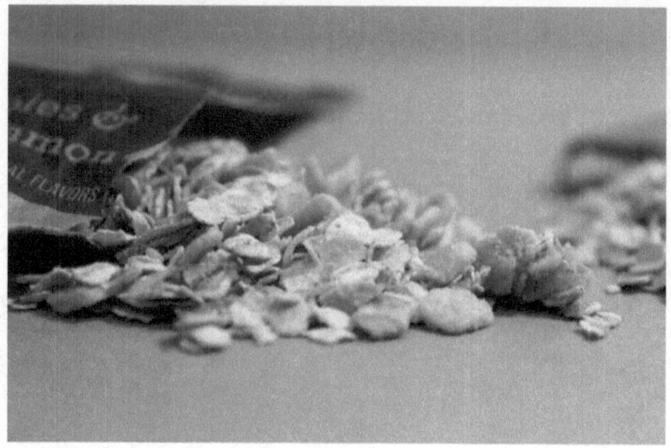

Ingredients:

- Organic essential oil
- Oatmeal.
- Cocoa powder
- Cinnamon.

Directions:

1. Mix the oatmeal or other base in a shaker container.

2. Sprinkle on scalp only by dividing hair sections using a comb. Then massage your scalp. The powder absorbs the oil from your scalp when you leave it on your hair for 5-10 minutes.

3. Brush your hair well until you cannot see the powder anymore.

DIY Organic Coconut and Honey Shampoo

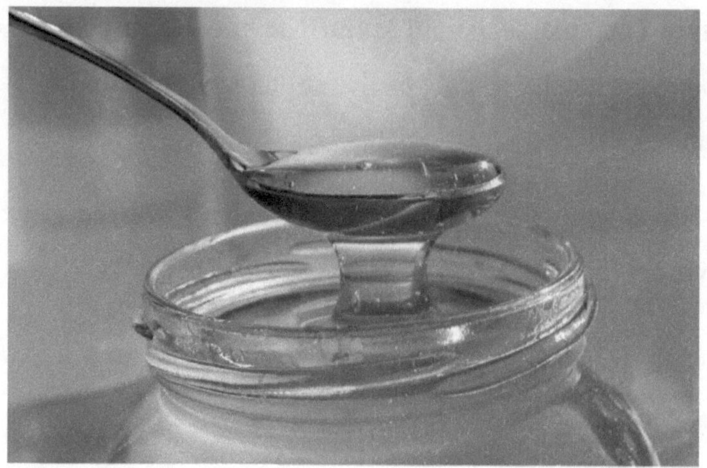

Ingredients:

- ¼ c. water, filtered
- ¼ tsp. organic rosemary essential oil
- Royal jelly
- ¼ c. organic liquid castile soap, unscented
- 1 c. organic coconut milk
- 2 tbsps. organic honey, raw
- 1 c. organic aloe-Vera gel

Directions:

1. Dissolve the honey in filtered warm water, no hotter than 100F.

2. Combine all other ingredients except for castile soup and blend them thoroughly.

3. Stir your castile soap in gently, using a whisk. Do not allow the soap to foam.

4. Pour the mixture into squirt bottles and store them in the refrigerator.

5. Before each use, shake the bottle well. You will see that the ingredients separate a bit, and this is OK.

6. Keep shampoo out of your eyes. If you do get some in the eyes, be sure to flush them right away with warm water.

DIY Organic Beer Shampoo!

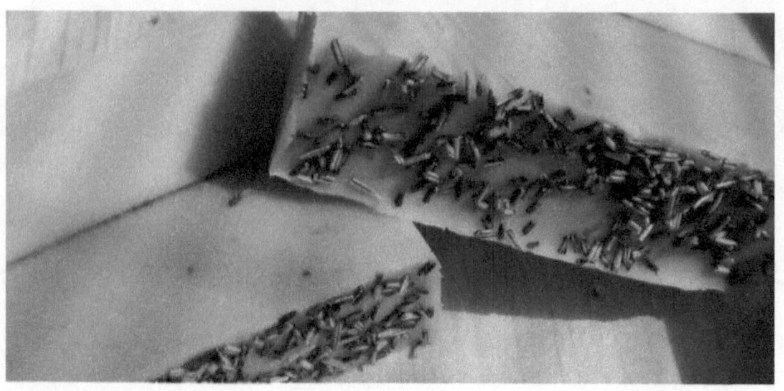

Ingredients:

- Organic shampoo
- 1 c. organic beer

Directions:

1. Measure one cup of organic beer from bottle or can. Put this in a pan without a lid. Heat over a medium high burner.

2. Boil beer for about 20 minutes or until it has been reduced to a half a cup or so.

3. Remove from heat and allow the beer to completely cool. This will take between five and 10 minutes.

4. Pour beer into organic shampoo and stir until well-blended. You may add or subtract your organic shampoo base amounts as you pour beer into it.

5. Use a funnel to transfer your DIY beer shampoo into a container with a secure lid.

6. Use this shampoo as you use any shampoo.

DIY Organic Baking Soda Shampoo

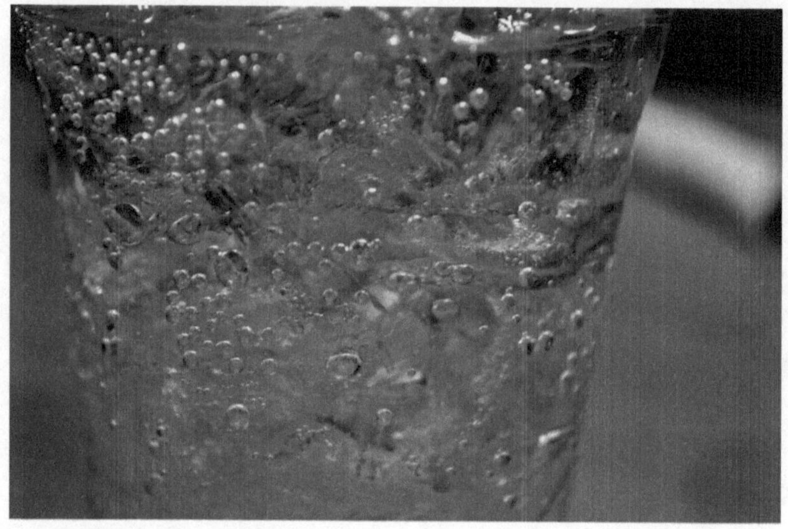

Ingredients:

- Warm water
- 2 tsps. baking soda

Directions:

1. Mix 2 teaspoons of baking soda into your water in a bowl. Pour gently over hair and massage. Rinse your hair thoroughly after you wash.

2. Repeat your rinse with a tablespoon of apple cider vinegar and water. This will ensure that all baking soda has been rinsed out.

DIY Organic Peppermint Bar Shampoo

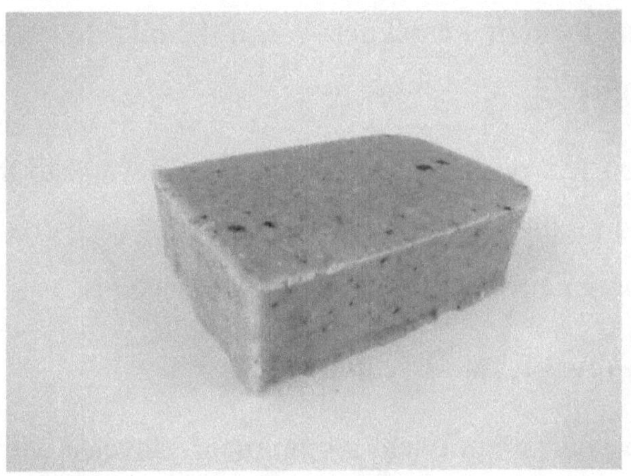

Ingredients:

- 10 oz. organic olive oil
- 12 oz. warm water, distilled
- 10 oz. organic coconut oil
- 1 ½ oz. organic peppermint essential oil
- 6 oz. organic castor oil
- 10 oz. organic palm oil

Directions:

1. Pour water into a bowl or jar.

2. Measure your oils, except for the essential oils, and combine them in a crockpot. Warm the oils slowly to 100-120 degrees F.

3. When you reach that temperature, add water to the oils. Blend until the mixture is fluid, but so that each drop of the mixture remains on the surface for 2-3 seconds.

4. Add your organic essential oils.

5. Pour your mixture into a soap mold. Cover it with a box turned upside down.

6. After about a day, remove the soap from your mold. Slice it. Stand your organic bars up and allow them to cure for about a month.

DIY Organic Olive Oil Shampoo

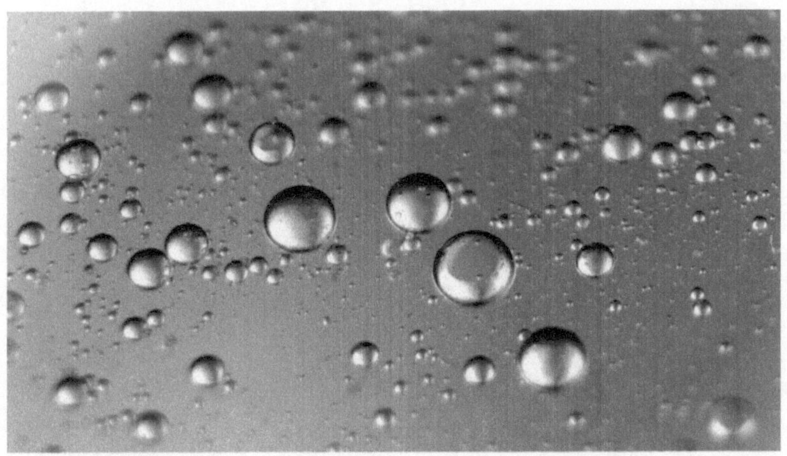

Ingredients:

- ½ c. warm water
- 1 c. organic castile soap
- Favorite organic essential oil
- ¼ c. organic olive oil

Directions:

1. Stir the ingredients all together. Pour into a bottle with a lid. Shampoo as you would with any conventional shampoo. Shake well before each use.

2. If you have oily hair, cut back a bit on the amount of olive oil in your recipe.

DIY Organic pH Balance Coconut Shampoo

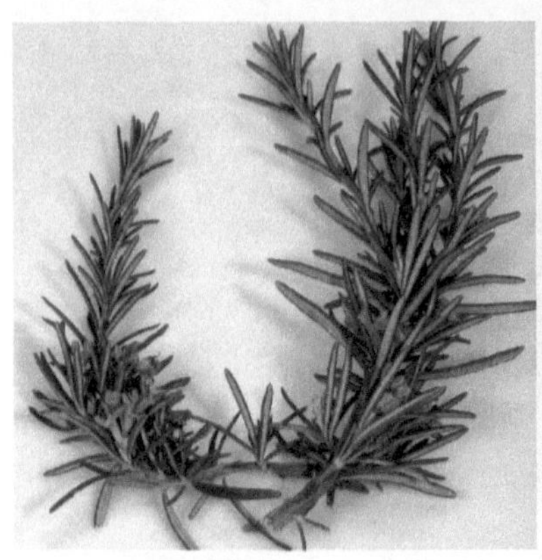 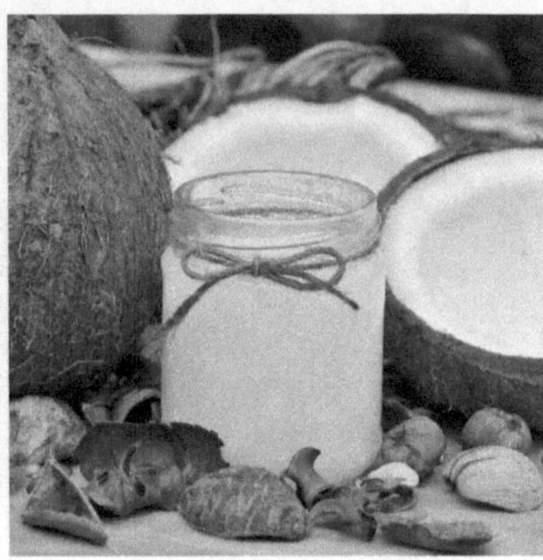

Ingredients:

- 1 tsp. organic jojoba oil
- 1 can fat coconut milk, organic
- 2 tbsps. organic apple cider vinegar
- 1 tsp. favorite organic essential oil
- 2 tbsps. organic raw honey
- 1 tsp. organic castor oil

Directions:

1. In a bowl, mix all ingredients. Whisk until the mixture is smooth.

2. To shampoo, massage a bit on your scalp and spread through your hair with a comb or your fingers. Leave shampoo on your hair for five minutes or so before you rinse.

3. If you have oily hair, you may do an organic apple cider rinse after this shampoo. Use 1/4 cup of water and 1/4 c. of organic apple cider vinegar.

DIY Organic Green Tea Shampoo

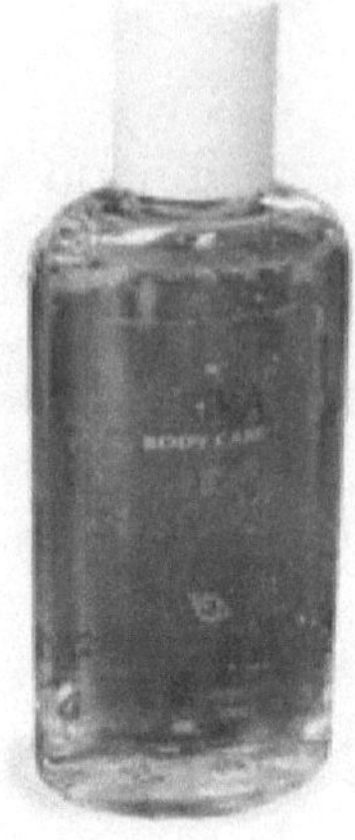

Ingredients:

- 1 tbsp. organic olive oil
- 1 c. organic castile soap, liquid
- 1 tbsp. organic honey, raw
- 1 c. organic green tea, brewed
- Sage leaves

Directions:

1. Mix the ingredients above and use as you would regular shampoo. You may also add an organic herbal infusion instead of green tea. In this case, you would use one spoonful of organic dried herbs and a cup of water and steep for a half hour.

Here are some optional ingredients to add, depending on your hair type:

To treat dandruff – burdock roots and nettle leaves

For treating normal hair – marigold flowers

To balance greasy hair – yarrow

For dark hair colors – sage leaves

Organic DIY Arrowroot Dry Shampoo

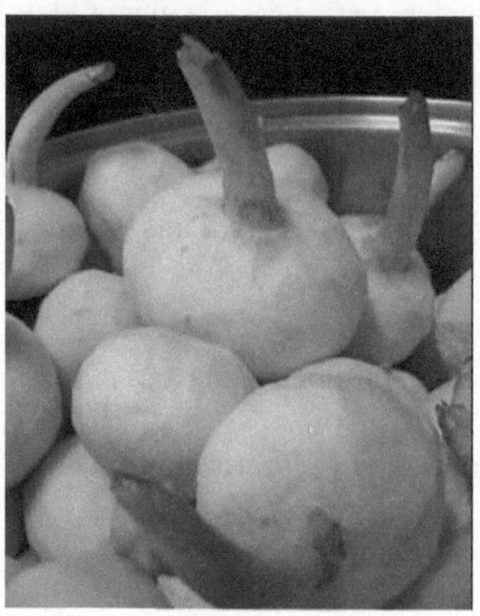

Ingredients:

- 1 c. organic arrowroot flour
- Few drops favorite organic essential oil

Directions:

2. Transfer your arrowroot flour into some type of container like a jar that has a lid. Add several drops of your favorite organic essential oils.

3. Apply to your hair roots with a clean makeup brush. Use a brush or comb to get to other scalp areas. Apply the powder in those areas, too. Once you have treated your scalp, brush out the majority of the powder and then style as usual.

Coconut Hot Oil Treatment for Normal Hair

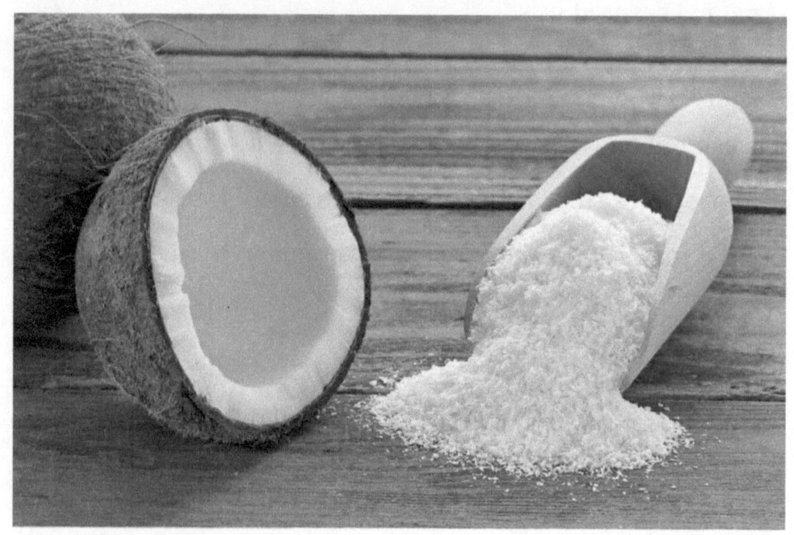

Ingredients:

- 24 drops Ylang Ylang oil
- 4 oz. coconut oil

Directions:

1. Over medium high heat, add water in a saucepan and allow to boil.

2. Reduce the heat to keep the water simmering.

3. Use 1% dilution, measure 24 drops of Ylang Ylang essential oil.

4. Mix the Ylang Ylang essential oil with 4 ounces of coconut oil in a heat proof container.

5. Place the heat proof container on the simmering water to infuse the oil.

6. Let the infused oil cool

7. Keep in an amber colored jar

DIY Homemade Hot Oil Treatment

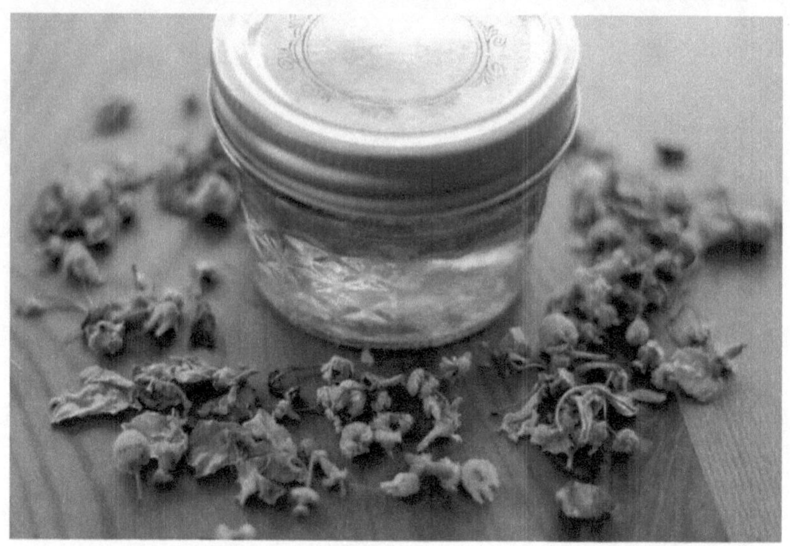

Ingredients:

- 2 small bunches rosemary, fresh
- 2 tbsps. avocado oil
- 8 drops peppermint essential oil
- 2 tbsps. olive oil
- 2 tsps. jojoba oil

Directions:

1. Boil water in a medium saucepan.

2. Reduce to low heat to simmer water.

3. Mix olive oil, avocado oil, jojoba oil in a heat proof bowl.

4. Add the fresh rosemary but make sure the herb is dry and has no moisture.

5. Place the heat proof bowl over the simmering water.

6. Infuse for 30 minutes.

7. Check constantly to avoid drying up.

8. After infusing the oil and the herb, let it cool a little, but make sure it is still warm when you add the peppermint.

9. Add the peppermint essential oil drops.

10. Transfer the infused oil in an airtight container.

Jojoba Hot Oil treatment for Frizzy Hair

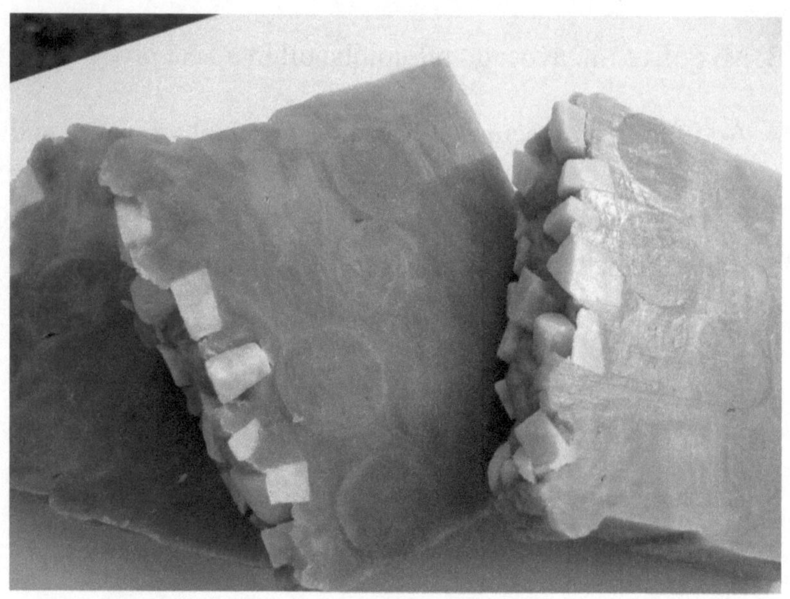

Ingredients:

- 2 tbsps. Argan oil
- 6 drops burdoch oil
- 2 tbsps. jojoba oil

Directions:

1. Boil hot water in a saucepan in high heat.

2. Reduce the heat to keep the water simmering.

3. Mix jojoba oil, argan oil and burdoch oil in a heatproof container.

4. Place the heat proof container on the simmering water to infuse the oil.

5. Let the infused oil cool.

6. Keep in an amber colored jar.

Creamy Coco oil deep conditioner

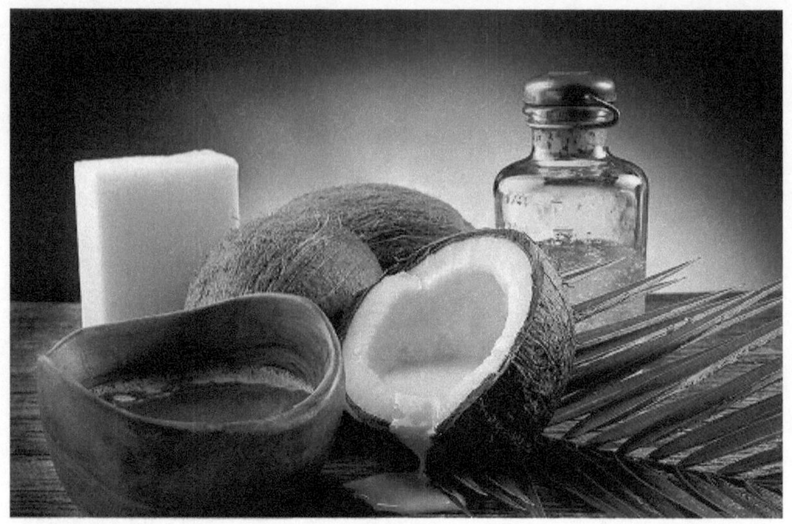

Ingredients:

- 1 tbsp. jojoba oil
- 5 drops Lavender essential oil
- 2 tbsps. coconut oil

Directions:

1. Solidify your coconut oil by leaving it in the fridge for a few minutes.

2. Take 2 tablespoons of solid coconut oil and stir it in a bowl until it melts into a creamy state.

3. Stir in the jojoba oil until well combined.

4. Stir in the drops of lavender essential oil to combine.

Coconut Oil deep hair conditioner

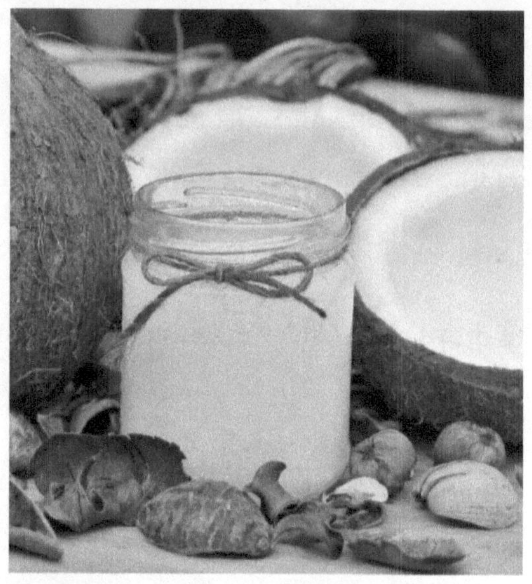

Ingredients:

- 8 drops Ylang Ylang essential oil
- 1 tbsp. olive oil
- Stand
- 3 tbsps. coconut oil

Directions:

1. Combine coconut oil, olive oil and essential oils in a mixing bowl.

2. Using a mixer, mix in medium/high speed all ingredients for 5 minutes or until the mixture becomes thick and creamy.

Coconut and Shea deep conditioner

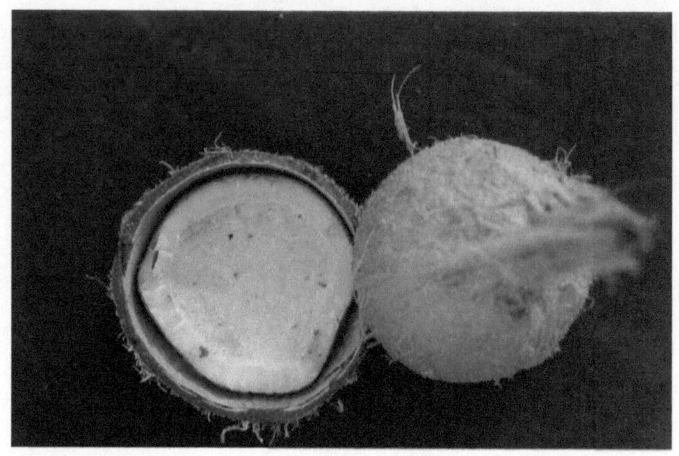

Ingredients:

- 3 drops Rosemary essential oil
- 1 tbsp. shea butter
- 1 tsp. argan oil
- 2 tbsps. coconut oil

Directions:

1. Measure coconut oil and shea butter in solid form.

2. Melt the solid form in a microwave or a double broiler.

3. Wait until the mixture cools and becomes creamy.

4. Add the argan oil and the drops of rosemary essential oil.

5. Whip for 3 minutes or until you get a creamy consistency.

Olive Oil Pre-Poo Hair Treatment

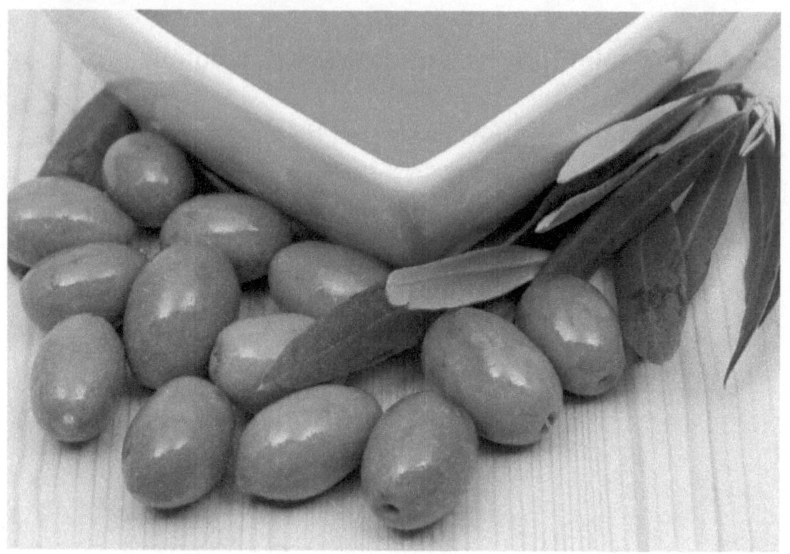

Ingredients:

- 4 drops tea tree essential oil
- ¼ c. Virgin olive oil
- 2 tbsps. castor oil

Directions:

1. Dilute tea tree essential oil with virgin olive oil and castor oil in a spritzer.

2. Mix and shake the oil mixture well.

Avocado Mask

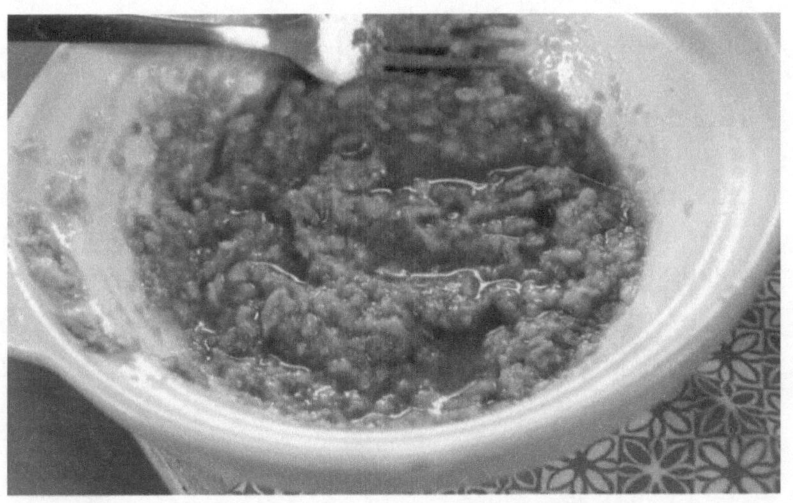

Ingredients:

- 1 tbsp. castor oil
- 1 tbsp. coconut oil
- 1 tbsp. olive oil
- 1 small avocado, ripe

Directions:

1. Mash the ripe avocado until it becomes thick and creamy in consistency.

2. Add the coconut, castor, and olive oils.

3. Mix until all the oil is blended.

4. (Optional) You can heat in low fire to make it thicker.

Pure carrier oil Pre Poo

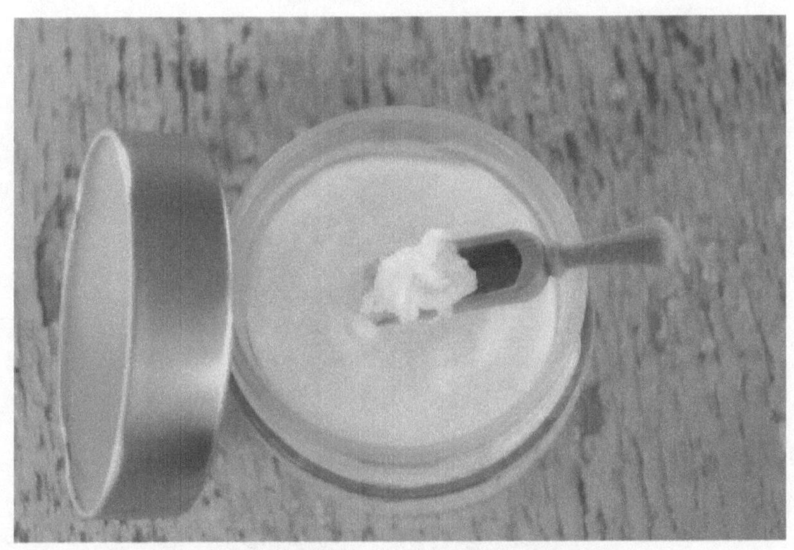

Ingredients:

- 2 tbsps. almond oil
- 2 tbsps. olive oil
- 2 tbsps. castor oil

Directions:

1. Mix the oils together in a spritzer.

2. Shake well.

Detangler leave in conditioner

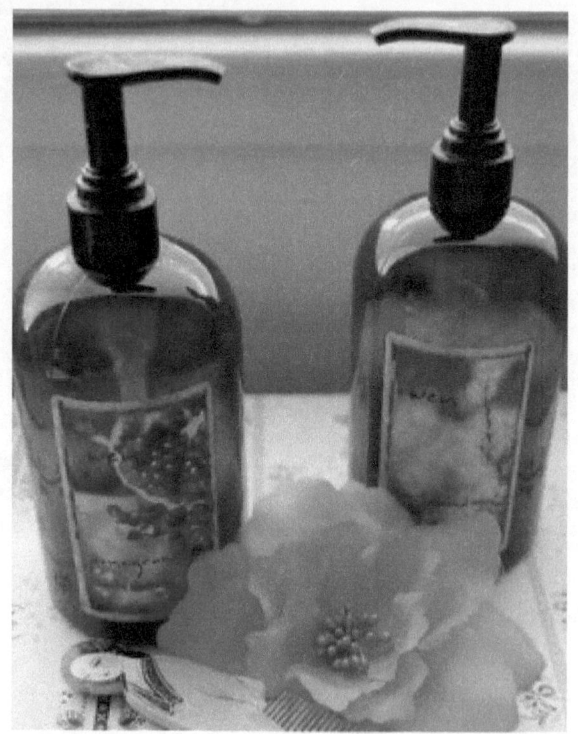

Ingredients:

- 1 tbsp. vegetable glycerin
- 10 drops rosemary essential oil
- 5 tbsps. distilled water
- 1 tbsp. aloe vera gel

Directions:

1. Place the aloe vera gel on a glass spray bottle.

2. Pour in the distilled water.

3. Add the vegetable glycerin.

4. Add the rosemary essential oil drops (you can also use lavender).

5. Cover the bottle and shake to mix until the aloe vera gel dissolves.

Creamy leave in conditioner

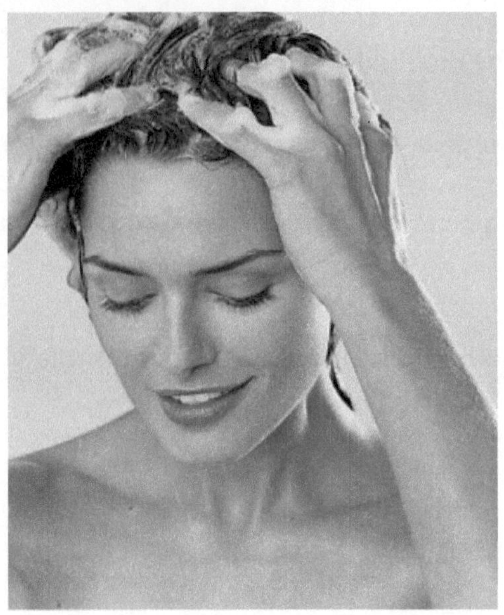

Ingredients:

- 2 oz. aloe vera gel
- 1 tsp. avocado oil
- 1 oz. coconut oil, softened

Directions:

1. Combine all ingredients in a mixing bowl.

2. Beat with an electric mixer until the consistency becomes thick and creamy.

Basic Shampoo Recipe

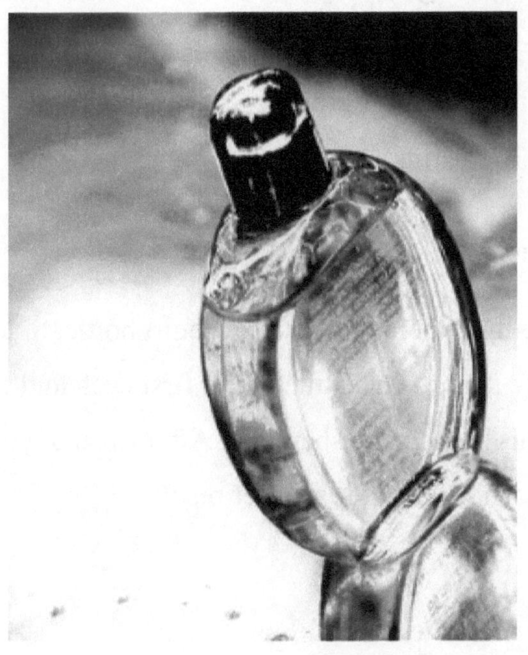

Ingredients:

- ½ tsp. vegetable glycerin
- ¼ tsp. vitamin E oil
- 2 tbsps. Aloe Vera gel
- ½ c. Castile Soap, liquid

Directions:

Put all the ingredients in a plastic squirt bottle. Shake well to mix. Make sure to shake the bottle first each and every time you use this homemade shampoo. After rinsing, you may use a natural conditioner for a softer result.

Herbal Shampoo

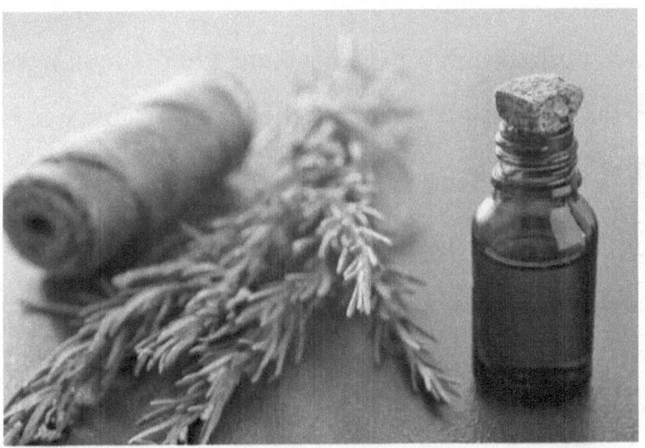

Ingredients:

- ½ tbsp. Grape seed oil
- ¼ c. water, distilled
- ¼ c. liquid castile soap
- 2 tbsps. tea oil
- ½ tbsp. vanilla extract
- 3 tbsps. rosemary

Directions:

1. Pour the distilled water into a pot and bring it to a boil.

2. When boiled, turn off the heat and add the lemongrass tea leaves and the rosemary. Strain the leaves from water and let it cool.

3. Add the rest of the ingredients into the pot and stir well. Transfer in a sealed bottle for use.

Coco Shampoo

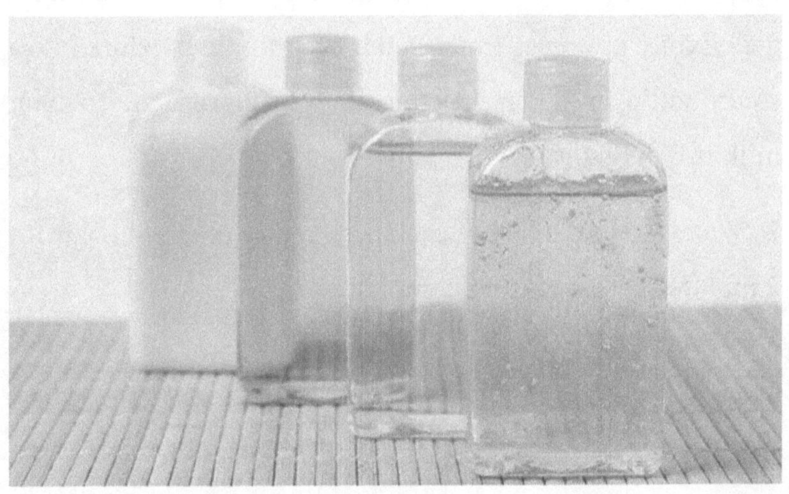

Ingredients:

- 1 tsp. castor oil

- 15 drops lavender essential oil

- 2/3 c. castile soap

- ½ c. coconut milk

- 1 tsp. sweet almond oil

Directions:

1. Mix all the ingredients in a bowl. Blend them well until the mixture produces frothy bubbles. Pour the mixture into a squirt bottle, and then shake again to make sure the coconut milk is blended well.

2. Shake the bottle before each use. Lather onto your hair for 2 minutes before rinsing completely.

Aloe Shampoo

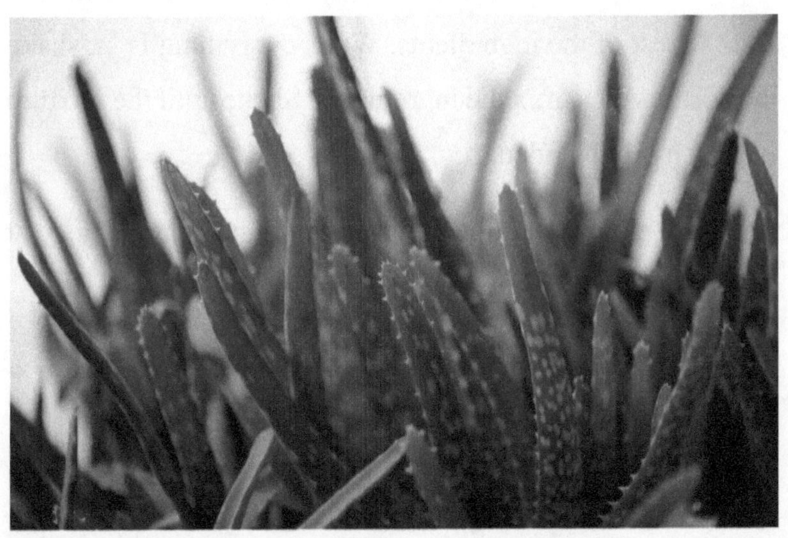

Ingredients:

- 1 tsp. vegetable glycerin
- ¼ c. liquid castile soap
- ¼ c. Aloe Vera gel
- ¼ tsp. olive oil

Directions:

1. Pour the liquid castile soap into a squirt bottle first then add the rest of the ingredients. When everything is in, shake the bottle well to mix the ingredients. Shake until the mixture is thoroughly blended.

2. To use, give the bottle a few shakes first and apply as you normally would shampoo.

Egg Shampoo

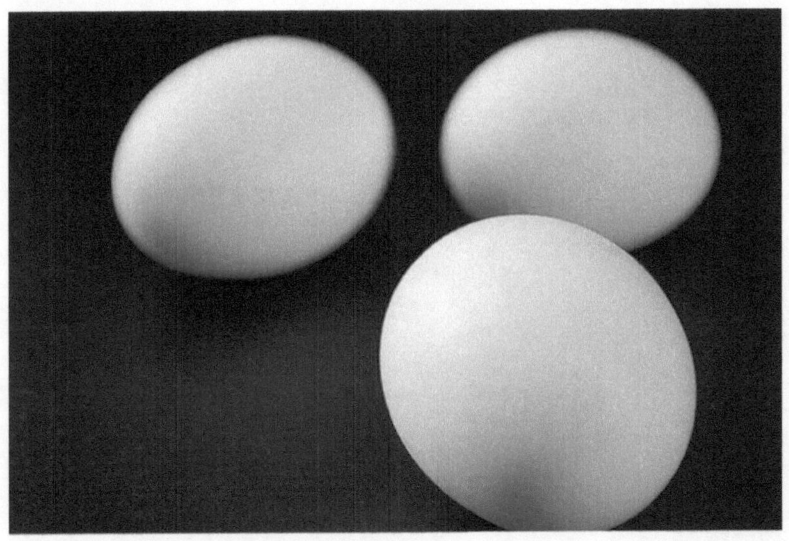

Ingredients:

- 1 tbsp. honey
- 2 tbsps. lemon juice, freshly squeezed
- 2 eggs, whole
- 3 drops olive oil

Directions:

1. In a bowl, mix all ingredients. Wet your hair with warm water from a spray bottle.

2. Apply the mixture evenly to hair.

3. Leave on for a good 2 minutes and rinse thoroughly with lukewarm water.

Banana Deep Conditioner

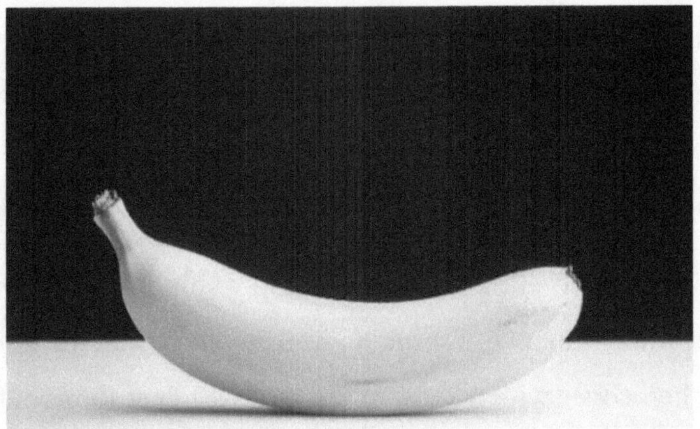

Ingredients:

- ¼ c. Greek yogurt
- 1 tbsps. honey, pure
- 1 whole peeled and sliced banana, ripe
- 2 tbsps. olive oil

Directions:

1. Process the sliced banana and extra virgin olive oil in a blender. Blend them until smooth. Pour the rest of the ingredients in and mix until the lumps and chunks are gone. Use a strainer to sift through the mixture. Pour your deep conditioning mixture through the strainer to a container.

2. To deep condition your hair, apply this mixture to wet hair. Make sure every strand is well covered from the root to tip then cover with a shower cap. Allow to set for about 30 mins and rinse completely.

Yogurt Deep Conditioner

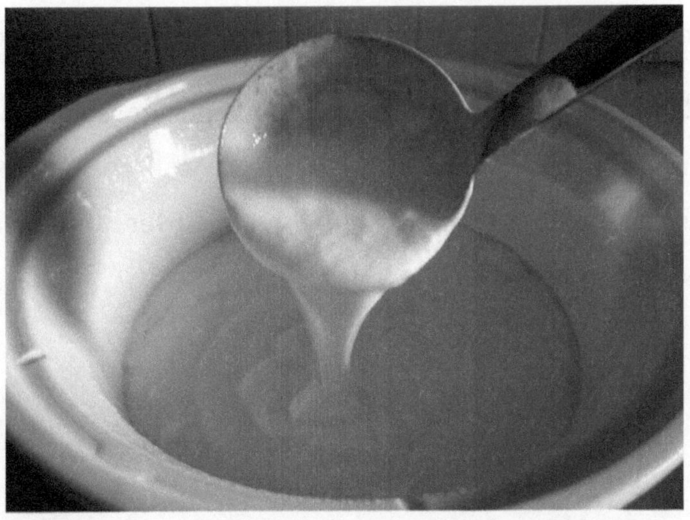

Ingredients:

- 1 tbsp. coconut oil
- 1 c. Greek yogurt
- 1 tbsp. castor oil
- 1 whole egg, whipped

Directions:

1. Pour the yogurt in a glass bowl and whip it well until smooth. Add the rest of the ingredients. Stir well to blend.

2. To use the deep conditioner, apply a generous amount to your damp hair. When every strand is well coated, cover your head with a shower cap. Allow to sit for 30 mins and rinse completely.

Mayo Deep Conditioner

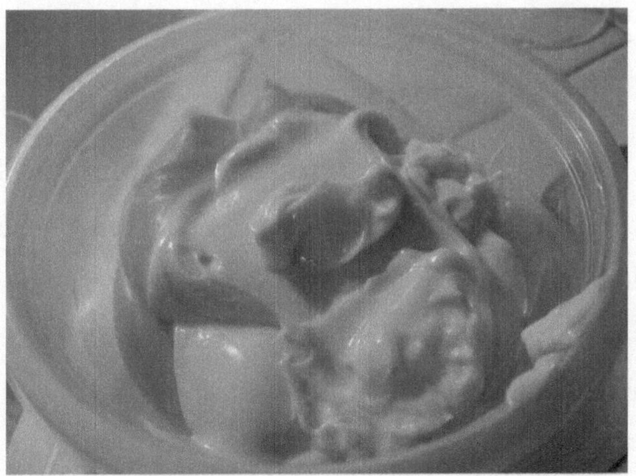

Ingredients:

- 1/3 c. yogurt, plain
- 2 tbsps. honey
- 1 c. mayonnaise
- 1/3 c. coconut oil

Directions:

1. In a bowl, add all ingredients. Whip them to mix together. Stir to obtain a smooth consistency and your deep conditioner is ready for use.

2. To use this homemade hair treatment recipe, apply the mixture liberally to your damp hair. You can separate your hair into sections to make sure it is evenly coated. Then, cover your head with a plastic cap. Allow to sit for 30 mins and rinse thoroughly.

Avocado Conditioner

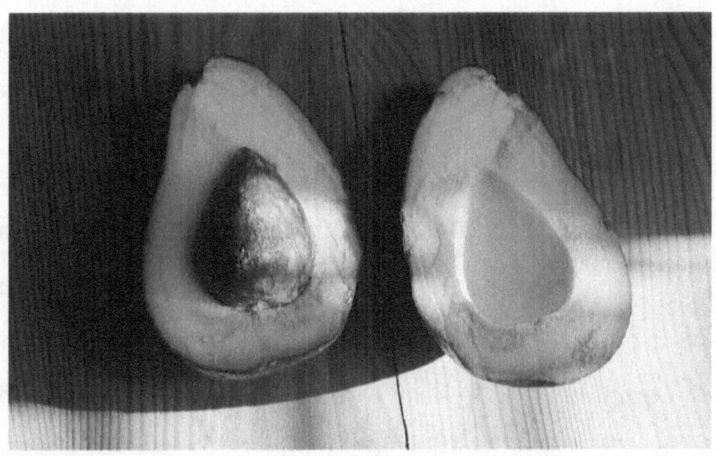

Ingredients:

- 1 tbsp. avocado oil
- 1 avocado, peeled and mashed
- 2 tbsps. organic honey

Directions:

1. Pour the mashed avocado along with the other ingredients in a blender. Process the ingredients until you have a smooth mixture.

2. Divide your hair into sections. Apply a generous amount of the mixture into each section until your hair is evenly coated. Your hair should be covered with a shower cap and leave it on for a whole hour. When the timer expires, rinse your completely. For best results, apply light conditioner after the deep conditioning treatment.

Sesame Deep Conditioner

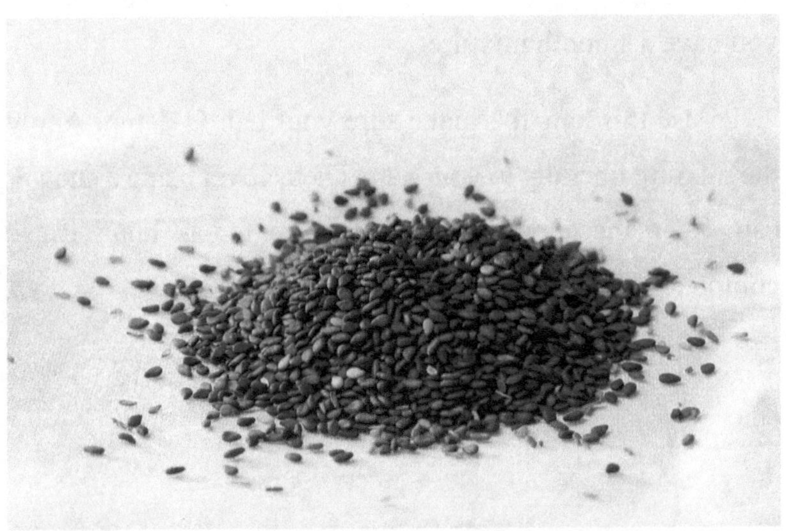

Ingredients:

- 2 tbsps. Aloe vera gel
- 1 tbsp. extra virgin olive oil
- 2 drops tea tree oil
- 1 c. Greek yogurt
- ¼ c. sesame seed oil

Directions:

1. In a bowl, add in all the ingredients. Whip them good until you have a smooth mixture.

2. To use this hair fix, make sure your hair is damp. Apply the mixture liberally to your hair. Then, cover using a shower cap. Keep the conditioner and cap on for an hour. Rinse completely.

Honey Coco Deep Conditioner

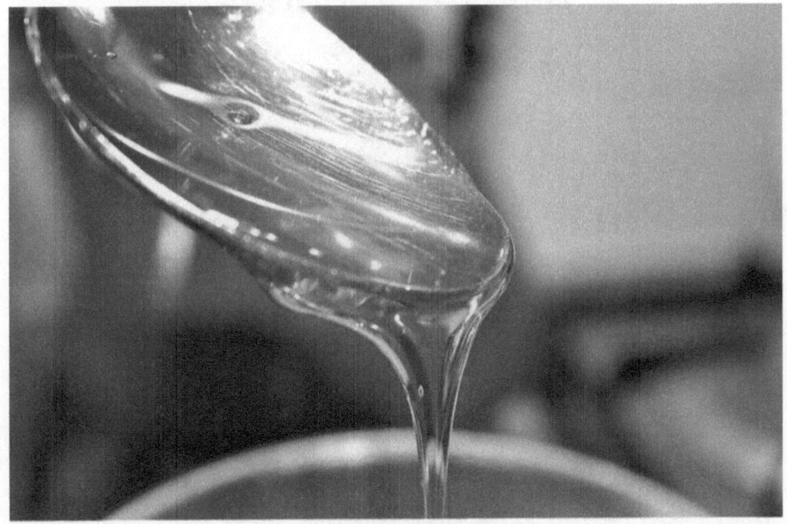

Ingredients:

- 3 tbsps. honey
- 6 tbsps. coconut oil

Directions:

1. Pour the ingredients in a glass bowl and stir together until well blended. Apply the mixture to your damp hair.

2. When your strands are well coated, cover your head with a plastic cap. Leave it on for 30 minutes up to 1 hour then rinse thoroughly.

Organic DIY Cider & Essential Oil Hair Conditioner

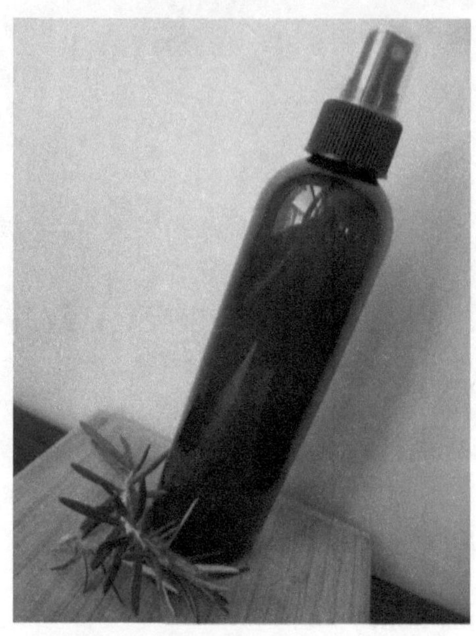

Ingredients:

- 12 drops of favorite organic essential oils
- 1 c. clear water
- 2 tbsps. organic apple cider vinegar

Directions:

1. Mix your ingredients in a spray bottle.

2. Shake well and then spray the conditioner on your hair.

3. Leave the conditioner in for five minutes and then rinse well.

The Simplest DIY Organic Hair Conditioner

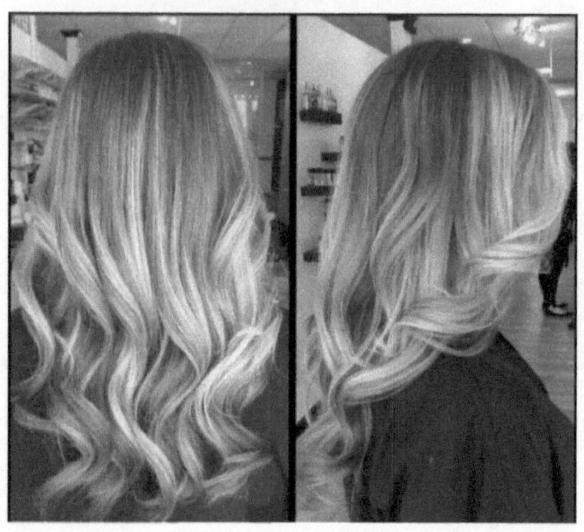

Ingredients:

- 1 c. water
- 1 tbsp. organic apple cider vinegar

Directions:

1. Combine the ingredients in a clean, re-used squirt bottle. To use, shake the bottle and massage the conditioner into your scalp and hair for a couple minutes. Then rinse well. After your hair dries, it won't retain the vinegar smell.

2. This simple organic conditioner works best after using a home-made organic shampoo. Whether you use baking soda or castile soap in your shampoo, this conditioner will smooth your hair and eliminate any sticky, greasy feeling the shampoos might leave.

Organic DIY Easy & Natural Hair Conditioner

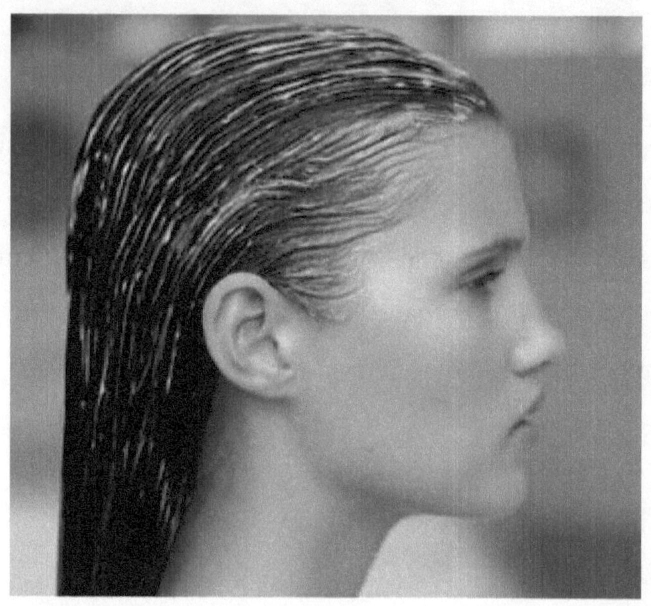

Ingredients:

- 1 tbsp. organic emulsifying wax
- ½ tsp. vitamin E
- ½ c. water, distilled
- 5 drops organic grapefruit seed extract
- 1 tsp. organic vegetable glycerin
- 1 tsp. almond oil

Directions:

1. Stir emulsifying wax, glycerin and oil in top of double boiler. Warm on slow heat until wax melts. Remove from stove and add vitamin E.

2. In another pot, warm water until it is only lukewarm. This step cannot be skipped, or the conditioner ingredients will become separated.

3. Pour water slowly in with oil mixture. Stir well with a whisk until consistency is smooth and creamy. Allow the mixture to cool a bit, so your essential oils won't evaporate quickly when they are added. It will not thicken immediately. This is normal. It will thicken as its temperature falls to the temperature in the room.

4. Stir in organic grapefruit seed extract and essential oils. Pour into a clean plastic bottle. Make sure it's cool before you put a lid on it.

5. Shake this bottle occasionally while conditioner is cooling, so that the ingredients won't separate.

Organic Lavender & Coconut Oil DIY Hair Conditioner

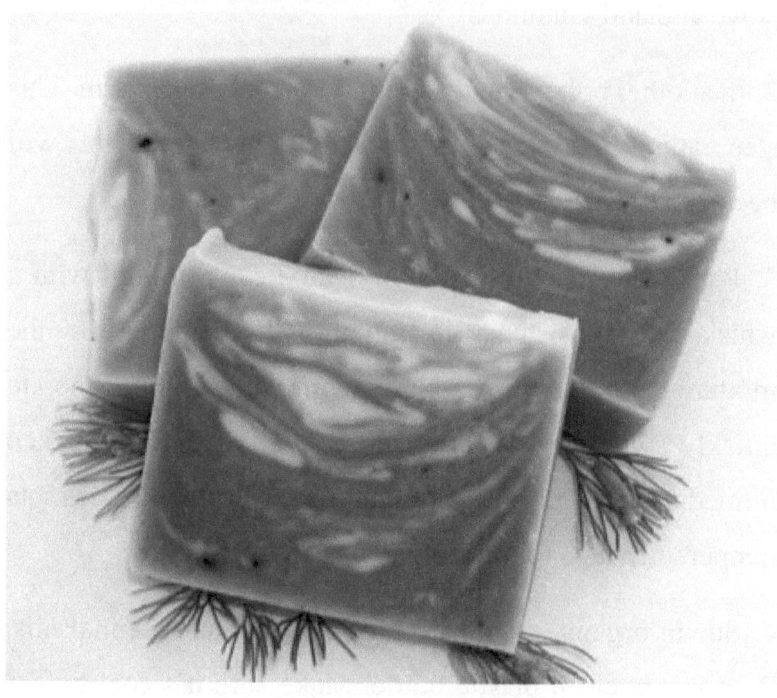

Ingredients:

- 1 tsp. organic vitamin E oil
- 1 tsp. organic jojoba oil
- 5 drops organic lavender essential oil
- 1 c. organic coconut oil

Directions:

1. Put all the ingredients in a clean pan.

2. Mix over high heat for 5-7 minutes.

3. Transfer into a plastic container when cooled.

4. Since coconut oil will melt in higher temperatures, if you live in a warm area, you can store this conditioner in your refrigerator. Or you can just use it as a liquid – it will still work. The mixture will remain fresh until the expiration date on the organic coconut oil.

5. Apply only a tiny conditioner amount to already-wet hair, after you have shampooed and rinsed. Start with the ends and work through all your hair. Avoid the top of the head.

Organic Honey & Aloe Vera DIY Hair Conditioner

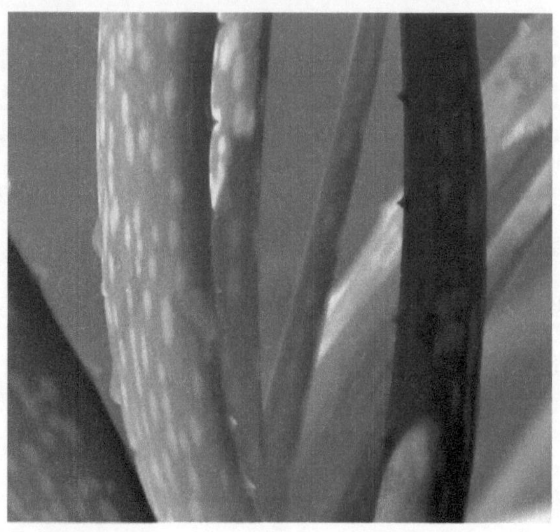

Ingredients:

- Organic aloe Vera gel
- Organic honey

Directions:

1. Mix organic honey and aloe Vera gel in equal parts. You can make small or large batches. Smaller batches work better if you don't use much of the product at any one time.

2. Massage mixture into hair.

3. Allow this conditioner to sir for 5-8 minutes.

4. Rinse your hair well.

Organic Olive Oil DIY Homemade Conditioner

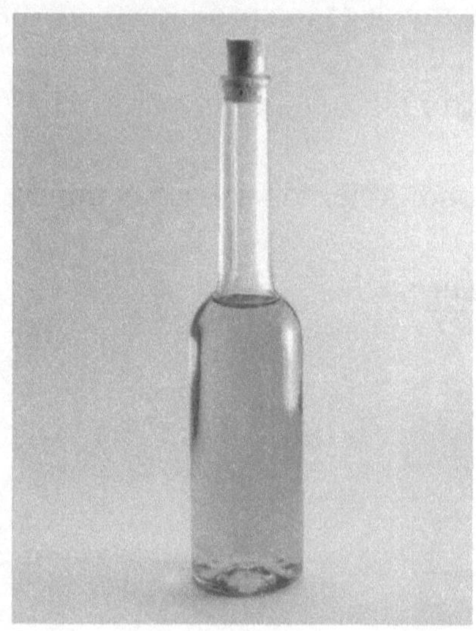

Ingredients:

- ¼ c. organic olive oil
- ½ c. organic regular DIY conditioner
- 5 drops any organic essential oil

Directions:

1. Combine DIY regular organic conditioner and olive oil in a medium bowl. Add essential oils and mix well.

2. Apply to your hair section by section.

3. Let sit for approximately 15 minutes or more.

4. Then detangle and fully rinse.

DIY Tropical Island Organic Hair Pre-Conditioner

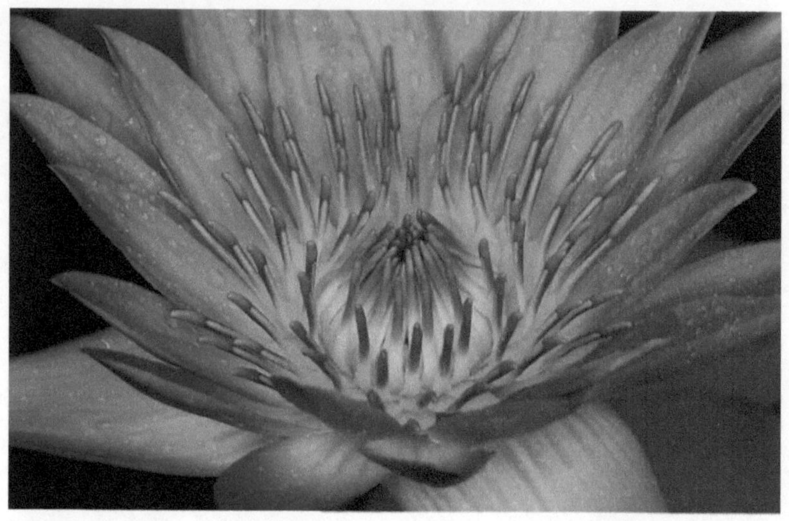

Ingredients:

- 1 avocado, organic
- 1 c. coconut milk, organic

Directions:

1. Peel the avocado and remove the pit. Mash well.

2. Add coconut milk slowly until the consistency is like that of commercial conditioner.

3. Use on hair from roots to ends.

4. After 15 minutes, rinse well and shampoo with DIY organic shampoo.

DIY Organic Herbal Hair Conditioner

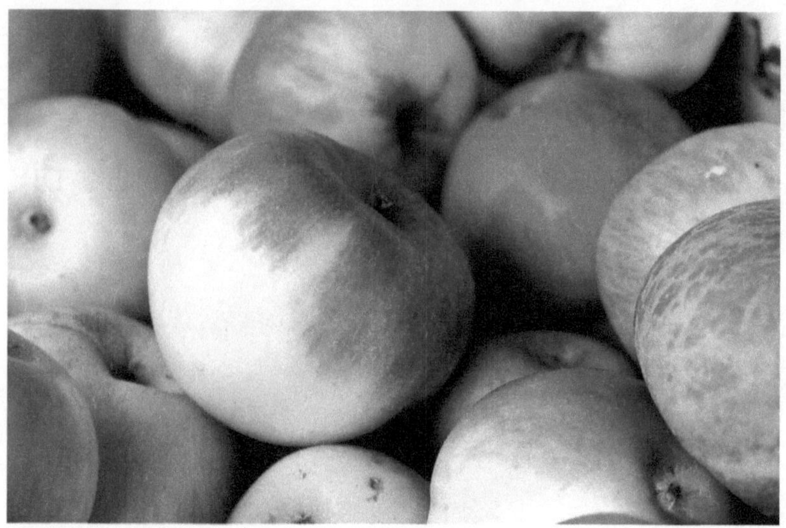

Ingredients:

- 2 tbsps. organic apple cider vinegar
- 3 tbsps. organic rosemary.
- 3 tbsps. lavender.
- 2 c. water, distilled
- 3 tbsps. organic peppermint
- 3 tbsps. chamomile

Directions:

1. Combine 2 cups of distilled water with your suitable herbs above.

2. Pour into a pot and boil on stove.

3. Remove from stove and allow to steep for one hour

4. Strain herbs out and pour remainder into clean plastic bottle.

5. Add the organic apple cider vinegar.

6. Mix well.

7. To use, pour over hair after it is conditioned. Rub gently into scalp and rinse.

DIY Rosemary & Herbal Tea Organic Hair Conditioner

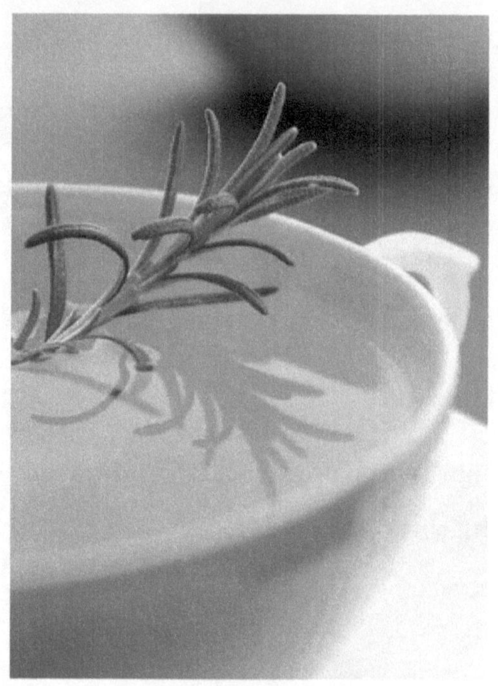

Ingredients:

- ¼ sprig organic rosemary
- 2 ½ c. water, hot
- ½ c. apple cider vinegar
- 1 bag herbal tea

Directions:

1. Pour water into a plastic bottle. You can re-use conditioner bottles if you like.

2. Add remaining ingredients.

3. Allow mixture to sit for one-half hour.

4. Shake bottle well before each use.

5. Use a little over 1/2 cup of conditioner after every shampoo.

DIY Organic Shea Butter & Aloe Hair Conditioner

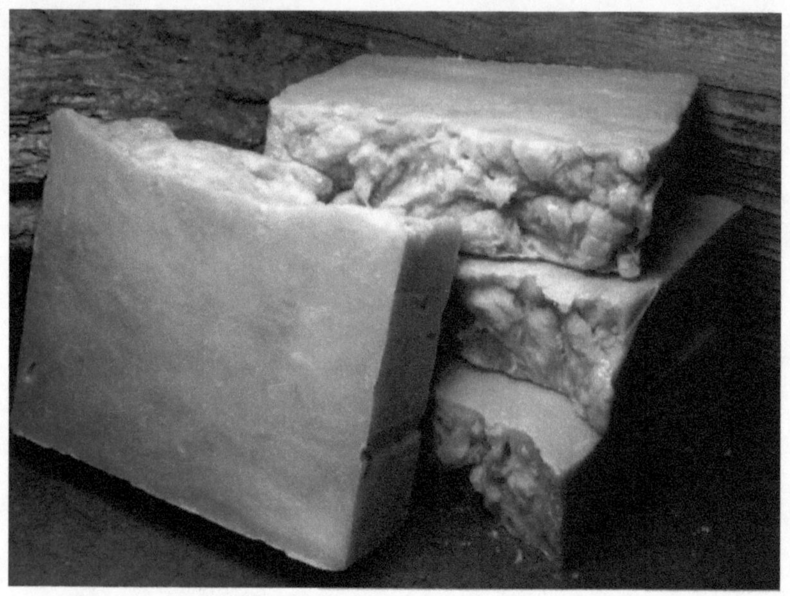

Ingredients:

- 1 tsp. organic safflower oil
- ¼ c. raw Shea butter
- ¼ c. organic soothing aloe Vera gel
- 2 tsps. organic grapeseed oil
- 6 drops organic lavender essential oil

Directions:

1. Soften Shea butter if it's hard – place in a heat-safe container and immerse in hot water.

2. Add organic safflower oil and organic grapeseed oil. Stir briskly or use a hand mixer to blend.

3. Add the organic aloe Vera gel and continue to whisk. Be sure the consistency is smooth.

4. Transfer your conditioner to a clean plastic container. Stir in your organic lavender essential oil.

5. Store in a place that is cool and dark.

Coco Deep Conditioner

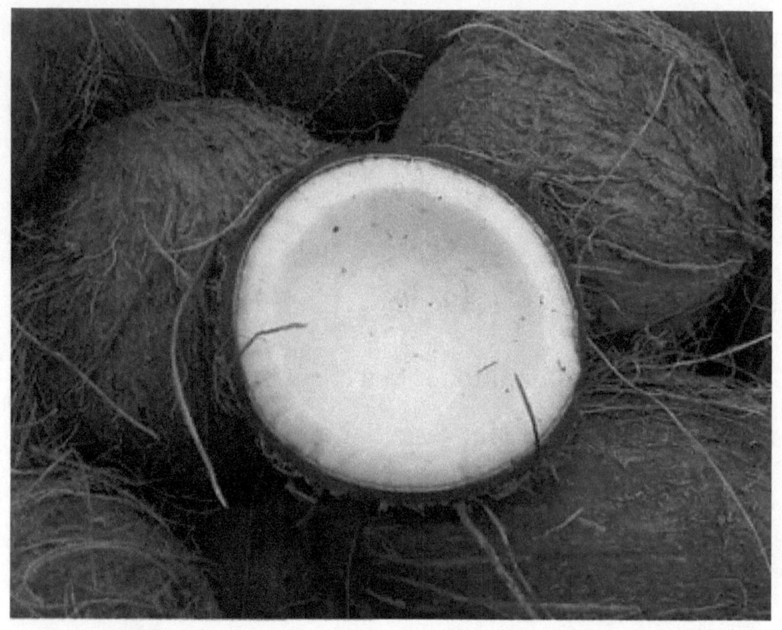

Ingredients:

- ½ c. honey
- ½ c. coconut milk, pure
- 1 ½ c. water, distilled
- 1 tbsp. coconut oil

Directions:

1. Set all ingredients in your food processor. Blend until smooth. Transfer the mixture to a saucepan and then heat until warm. It should only be heated enough for your fingers to handle. Avoid overheating it.

2. Once ready, apply the mixture to your damp hair. To make sure it is evenly coated, divide your hair into sections. Apply a generous amount to each section.

3. Once your hair is coated evenly from root to tip, cover your head with a shower cap. Leave it on for 30 minutes up to 1 hour or more if you have the time. The longer you leave this deep conditioner on your hair, the softer each strand will get.

Conclusion

You have what it takes to take great care of your hair so that you can enjoy all the incredible benefits it will bring you! Be sure to start right now and get started with a few of the recipes and tips in this book. If one doesn't work for you, another will, so just keep experimenting with these options until you find your perfect hair care solution.

You won't always get a healthy, strong, colorful, and full head of hair by overwhelming it with the chemicals found in commercial products. However, you now have a balanced array of natural hair product recipes from which to choose. There's no need to use them all at once; just select what your type of hair needs most and start there.

Maintaining a healthy head of hair is your best defense against dull and lifeless hair, thinning hair, and baldness. While you can't prevent hereditary hair loss, you can slow it by using the incredible recipes and advice in this book. Remember that some of these suggestions may not work if you have chemically straightened or curled hair and some may wash out any commercial coloring you've added. Don't be afraid to experiment a little bit and then enjoy your radiant and beautiful hair!

Author's Afterthoughts

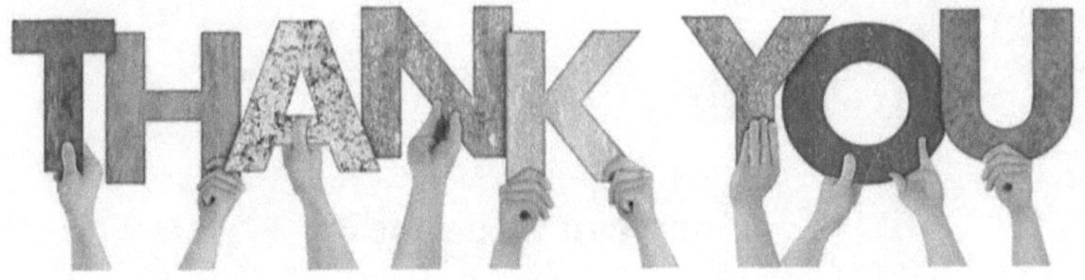

With so many books out there to choose from, I want to thank you for choosing this one and taking precious time out of your life to buy and read my work. Readers like you are the reason I take such passion in creating these books.

It is with gratitude and humility that I express how honored I am to become a part of your life and I hope that you take the same pleasure in reading this book as I did in writing it.

Can I ask one small favour? I ask that you write an honest and open review on Amazon of what you thought of the book. This will help other readers make an informed choice on whether to buy this book.

My sincerest thanks,

Angel Burns

If you want to be the first to know about news, new books,
events and giveaways, subscribe to my newsletter by
clicking the link below

https://angel-burns.gr8.com

or Scan QR-code